Holistic Self-Healing #1

Start Healing
with
Positive Thinking

Mastering Positive Thinking,
Improving Immunity,
Becoming Healthier Now!

By

Dr. Lloyd Stenbeck

By Dr. Stenbeck

Books

Healing Yourself -- The Holistic Approach
Heal Yourself Right Now!

The 22 Unique Body Types! *(Thin, Muscle, Fat)*
   -- with separate volumes in preparation on the
     22 Types:
      - The Six Thin Body Types
      - The Nine Muscle Body Types
      - The Seven Fat Body Types
      - Booklets on each of the 22 Body Types

Booklets
(Concise step-by-step details on accomplishing each issue)

#1 Start Healing with Positive Thinking
#2 Mastering Positive Feelings for Health
#3 Spiritual Balance and Your Healing

Library of Congress Catalog Card Number:

TXU 127-897

Disclaimer

The philosophy, causes of illness, and methods of healing presented here represent a holistic approach to your healing, adjunctive to and not a substitute for, medical diagnosis and the drug treatment of disease. Common sense dictates that you have a medical work-up before embracing any natural healing method. In healing yourself, it is important to remember that these booklets are not about clinical disease, which requires medical supervision. Do not stop taking medication without first consulting with your physician.

The booklets are about *sub*-clinical healing and those aspects of your healing that you have command over, namely your diet, nutrition, mental, emotional, and spiritual balance. These aspects are often keys to helping your body heal itself, even if diseased.

The publisher accepts no responsibility for any misuse of the information in this book—it is not a substitute for medication or for the appropriate medical care of a disease.

About the Author

Educated in New Zealand and in the U.S.A., Dr. Stenbeck attained B.S., M.S., D.C. degrees. His holistic healing methods have been profiled in magazines (Esquire, McLean's, Playgirl, the Atlanta Constitution), and on TV in the USA and in Canada. He was the main contributor to the Warner Book *The Eye/Body Connection* by Jessica Maxwell, focusing on holistic healing relationships between the iris and organ genetics.

In the 1970-80's he was elected Fellow, Royal Society of Health, London; Fellow, American Association of Chemists; Member, American Association of Clinical Chemists; and Affiliate, Royal Society of Medicine, London. He studied naturopathy and Body Types with Dr. Bernard Jensen and Dr. Clifford Severn, and has practiced in clinics where patients received the joint benefits of medical and holistic healing.

His personal healing agenda includes subjects not mentioned here such as exercise, detoxifying diets, and periodic juice fasting with protein drinks. He is semi-retired, and a member of Self-Realization Fellowship. To receive complimentary holistic advice on any one health issue, see his web site: *DrStenbeck.net*

Contents

You may need behavioral changes
to lessen your mental stress and
to enhance your healing.

Adrenal hypoglycemia (low blood sugar)
must be resolved since it causes
more mental stress.

You may have a DNA or life lesson
factor causing mental stress and
interfering with your healing.

Symptoms of Mental Stress

Mental stress internalized in organs causes these common symptoms, first confirmed by the extensive research of the famous physician and scientist, Hans Selyē, M.D., Ph.D.

Fatigue, failure to heal, unable to think positively, having a "runaway mind", lymphatic congestion, immune problems, infections, moods/ depression (not clinical), migraines; head, neck, mid-back pain; adrenal hypoglycemia, low blood sugar, stomach-intestinal irritation, ulcers, and negative or neurotic thinking.

From this list, you will appreciate the amount of healing that depends on you mastering the mental stress of life.

* * *

Introduction

This series of succinct booklets provides more specific, step-by-step instructions, on proceeding with your healing. They are a logical follow-up to the earlier books on holistic self-healing:

Healing Yourself -- The Holistic Approach.

This book provides you with a selection of subjects covering common physical problems and personal growth issues. It is an excellent introduction to this healing, and to the tool of muscle testing.

Heal Yourself Right Now!

This book is a detailed walk-through every organ in the body and how to help yourself from the mental, emotional, spiritual, diet, and nutritional supplement perspectives. If interested in healing yourself, I strongly recommend you dig est these two books.

* * *

Muscle Testing

Muscle testing is a method of asking your mind how to proceed in your healing with the highest probability of success. If efficient with this tool use it in this booklet to confirm your choices for accomplishing positive thinking and healing. You make excellent progress *without* doing this testing, but it does give you an edge. (My previous books describe doing this test.)

▶ *The findings presented in this booklet are based on the clinical healing of patients using muscle testing (Applied Kinesiology), where your mind suggests healing priorities to the doctor.*

Your mind (higher self, innate intelligence, etc.), with high probability communicates a therapeutic approach to your healing, which after application enriches your health and promotes disease prevention (see previous books).

▶ *If you desire a more competent testing ability or want to learn more about this technique, take one of the internationally available* <u>*Touch for Health*</u> *courses for lay people.*

* * *

Use Your Common Sense

It should be obvious that any organ requiring medical attention must be cared-for before attempting any form of holistic healing. Working with a doctor who identifies your exact mental, emotional, and spiritual issues always magnifies healing; but such doctors are somewhat difficult to find, hence the existence of these booklets. (See *Appendix* for information on finding Health doctors.)

* * *

Mastering Mental Stress

This present booklet provides the facts on overcoming negative thinking without the case histories and other data in the earlier books: just the facts. You will understand the steps to attaining positive thinking, recovering from negative thinking or a "runaway mind", and preventing stress retention from making you sick. Attaining mental balance is relatively easy and necessary for your healing.

Taking drugs may help you mentally, but I am talking about healing yourself naturally. Without mental balance and positive thinking, you *automatically* internalize mental stress into different organs, guaranteeing that you cannot heal anything. Medication will get you through the day, allow you to feel a bit better, but it is a temporary fix. Believe that you can heal yourself.

Mental balance is essential for disease prevention, but a caution for those of you with clinical depression, psychological problems, or who are on medication; when the brain or mental problem is in your family DNA, medication may well be essential for your brain to function as well as it now does. *[See Step 7]*

If medication helps you, then a nutritional or holistic approach may achieve little, although your health will still benefit from working through this booklet. Specifically, the information here is for those of you suffering with the challenges of everyday life, trying to get through the day and to stay on top of all your challenges.

Of course, you won't have all the following symptoms, but as your mental body heals you become more positive about your life, more positive about resolving present stresses, and more positive about creating the future you want—and you become healthier.

Hand Selye, M.D., Ph.D.

- Stages of Stress -

Stage One: Alarm

Stomach irritation, indigestion, low blood sugar, mood swings, fatigue, pallor, sweats, sugar craving

Stage Two: Resistance

Fatigue, salt craving, stomach hydrochloric acid deficiency, stomach and intestine irritation (or ulcer), adrenal gland exhaustion, thymus atrophy, lymph congestion

Stage Three: Exhaustion

Collapse, and potentially, death

[This Chart shows Selye's research findings, which parallel muscle testing findings.]

I recommend that you keep taking prescribed medication and not to ignore medical advice. If ever diseased, I will be first to consult a medical physician to understand the full medical implications of my condition. I would then consider how to proceed with my healing by utilizing both medical and holistic data. When that day comes, I choose to be "the healthiest person in the graveyard!"

The mental body is the first key to all natural or holistic healing.

* * *

* * *

Note that we all undergo mental and emotional stress in our lives. Mental refers to negative thinking, while emotional refers to unconscious feelings like anger, hate, sadness, humiliated, etc. Treat them separately for effective healing. (Our organs also internalize spiritual stress. See Booklet #3).

* * *

Step 1 — Mental Nutrition

Nutrition is essential to nurture a stressed nervous system and to start your healing.

* * *

Attaining mental balance and positive thinking is impossible without first taking command of your nutrition. Your diet should be low in processed foods, moderate in protein, and rich in raw fruits and vegetables. Follow this advice for a few months until you achieve mental balance and positive thinking, and then continue to eat healthier foods. For your holistic healing, avoid eating junk foods and do the following:

- Minimize or stop eating all foods and products containing white sugar, corn syrup, and chemical sweeteners.
- Eat plenty of salads, vegetables, whole grains, seeds, and nuts; eat three meals daily even if that is unusual for you.
- Have moderate protein, 3-4 oz., twice daily (eggs, fish, poultry, meat); or if vegetarian, have 20 gm. daily of a protein drink/shake, in addition to other vegetable protein foods that you eat.

Nutritional Supplements

It is essential to take nutritional supplements to nurture the nerves responsible for your thinking, as differentiated from other nutrition for brain and central nervous system function (see my earlier books).

Take the following nutritional supplements, two capsules of each, twice daily with food, for one month; then take them once daily for another month:

- Multi-Mineral Complex: the product should contain potassium, calcium, magnesium, zinc, etc. (in measurable amounts); capsules are preferred for ease of digestion. Do NOT take a trace mineral complex or a liquid mineral source to accomplish this healing—it will not work for this purpose.
- B-complex (measurable amounts of B-vitamins are needed, preferably at about 50-100 mg. strength).
- Chamomile or Chickweed herb (if you prefer a herbal tincture, take one dropper-full, twice daily, before meals. This is for nerve detoxifying of environmental metals and chemicals.)

Important

Continue taking these supplements until you complete the Steps, feel more mentally positive, and are expecting good things to happen in your life. You will not get well without this nutritional component in place. If you have an on-going stress condition, continue taking the nutrition once daily after completing all the Steps.

If you have discomfort or an allergic reaction to any supplement, always stop taking it, or try another source of the product. Allergies are common.

*** * ***

Notes and Questions

(A muscle test is helpful if you know that tool. Otherwise, use your intuition and best educated guess.)

* * *

1. Ask: Am I eating the right foods for healthy nerve function and positive thinking? What else do I need to eat (or not eat)?

_____

Need to Eat -

_____

_____

_____

Stop Eating -

_____

_____

_____

* * *

2. *Ask: Do I have continuing mental stress in my workplace or in a relationship?*

If so, you will need nutritional maintenance to handle that stress; continue taking one of the above supplements, once daily. Multi-minerals would be the best choice. If your stress is severe, everyday, continue taking all of the prior nutritional supplements! Be sure that you do the following *Step 2.*

_____

_____

_____

* * *

3. *Other thoughts around this issue*

_____

_____

_____

* * *

Step 2 — Mental Affirmations

Affirmations reinforce your positive thinking and healing.

* * *

Now that the nutrition is in place, it is often essential that you design an affirmation directing your conscious mind to be positive about your main worry. (If you remain negative, then mental stress overloads into the body causing health problems.)

You affirm by speaking out-loud to yourself a phrase that cancels or neutralizes a major worry. After two weeks, you start believing that what you are affirming is possible although a stronger affirmation may then be appropriate.

Doing the Affirmation

▶ *Speak the affirmation, twenty-one times, twice daily, for two weeks.*

Less repetition does not work; more is unnecessary. Only affirm things that are theoretically possible and that directly relate to your life.

* * *

Several things may worry you incessantly, potentially leading to stomach, adrenal, and immune problems. Believe that stopping mental stress-overloading into your body is possible.

The affirmation is always about your most important concern, the one causing most negative thinking, commonly:

- A financial struggle
- A relationship or work-related problem
- A painful family situation, or other worry

* * *

Affirmation Examples

"I choose to stay positive around _____."

"I manage my stresses and live in the moment."

"I accept that my life is stressful, and I choose to be happy anyway."

"I problem-solve my stress of _____ (person, finances, situation, etc.)"

"I become non-reactive to my (partner's, lover's, etc.) negativity as I live in the moment."

"My gratitude, blessings, and happiness come from living in the moment."

* * *

God in Affirmations

If appropriate for your belief systems, the affirmations are more effective if you include God (creator, universe, etc.) in them. Choose one or two that appeal to you:

"I surrender all my _____stress to God."

"God and I co-create my happiness as I live in the moment."

"God and I co-create mastery over my stress as I live in the moment."

"God and I co-create my staying positive in work (or in a relationship, project, etc.)."

"I am not my body or mind, I am spirit, and God is within me."

"I express gratitude and love to God for the blessings of my everyday life."

"I choose to believe God directs my life."

"I invoke divine patience and master my stress."

"I invoke divine patience as I become non-reactive to _____ ."

"Everything in my life is in divine perfect timing for my evolution."

* * *

Affirmations in Relationship Problems

"I will talk to my loved one everyday about resolving our relationship stress."

"I will seek counseling for us if the problem does not improve after __ weeks."

"I will do everything in my power to work out this problem and create my own happiness."

"If he/she refuses help, I will seek counseling for myself accepting that I have done my best to resolve the problem."

"I will not be used, owned, intimidated, controlled, or abused by my partner, or by anyone else, and will immediately work to remove myself from any abusive situation."

(Address other examples involving a boss, family, friends, etc., in a similar way. Don't do more than 2-3 affirmations daily. It will only confuse your mind.)

* * *

Inappropriate Affirmations

The following affirmations are *not* helpful, as they are too general and non-specific:

"I now attract my most perfect mate who brings me happiness and fulfillment."

[Better: "I am open to attracting a perfect mate, in divine perfect timing, for my highest evolution."]

"I now receive unlimited abundance, prosperity, and wealth."

[Better: "I now receive, in divine perfect timing, my abundance as a beloved son (or daughter) of God, as I master my life lessons."]

Spoken affirmations heal the mental body; *writing* about issues heals the emotional body (see Booklet #2).

* * *

Notes and Questions

(A muscle test is helpful if you know that tool. Otherwise, use your intuition and best educated guess.)

* * *

1. Ask: Do I need affirmations to help attain positive thinking and mental balance in my life?

If you feel stressed, affirmations are essential for your progress. Most affirmations start with: "I am..., I will..., I now..., I become..., I master..., I manage..., God and I co-create..., God and I become...."

Start constructing your affirmations here, about *money, job, relationship, family, etc., or something else?*

Affirmation #1 —

_____

_____

_____

Affirmation #2 —

_____

_____

_____

Affirmation #3 —

_____

_____

* * *

2. Other Thoughts

_____

_____

_____

* * *

Step 3 — Emotional Overloading into the Mental Body

Intense emotions overload into your mental body causing negative thinking and delayed healing.

* * *

This important aspect of releasing negative emotions (presented in the earlier books, and more detailed in Booklet #2) gives a deeper understanding of emotional healing. Re-visited here, this aspect is also important in mental body healing. Intense negative feelings may cause negative thinking or a "runaway mind" where your negative thoughts run wild creating scenarios of failure and ruin.

▶ *If these intense emotions are not released from your whole being, they overload into your mental body causing mental stress and negative thinking.*

What emotions bother you the most? Everyday feelings like anger, rage, fear, dread, etc., retained in specific organs, may overload into your mental body, but usually more intense feelings are involved. Eventually, potentially, this results in physical health problems of ulcers, hypoglycemia, and immune problems.

Common examples of such intense feelings:

- Ruined
- Destitute
- Humbled
- Ashamed
- Desperate
- Decimated
- Humiliated
- Obliterated
- Dishonored
- I'm a nobody
- My life is over
- Overwhelmed
- I'm a total failure
- Fear, dread, terror
- I will never get well
- Unreal expectations
- I might as well be dead
- God doesn't care for me
- There is no hope for me
- God will never embrace me
- I've made too many mistakes
- I have created a life of poverty
- God will never forgive my sins
- Perverted, defiled, sexual abuse

You are highly stressed if you own such feelings or some other intense emotion. Think about the circumstances that caused them and use the following written release to start accomplishing your mental balance, positive thinking, and healing.

Identify those extremely stressful feelings that overwhelmed you now or in the past. Such pain could have happened at any time from about age three onwards. Have an educated guess at your probable programming; even if incorrect you will still help your healing. Intent is the key.

* * *

The following written release of negative feelings is somewhat related to the release done in the *Twelve Step* programs, with some extra steps. It is a very efficient way to manage and reprogram your emotions, and psychologists I know find it very helpful in their practices.

[Note: If you have cuss words in your mind about someone or a situation, be sure to write them out or the reprogramming will not occur. In most cases, the release is done only once. Write as much as you need to get your story out: a few paragraphs, or pages, as is necessary.]

* * *

The Written Emotional Release

Part A: *I write about my pain with...*

Part B: *I now release the unconscious negative emotion, belief, etc., of feeling (anger, rage, etc.):*
Due to: _____*(name of person, event)*
Age (about): _____*(or my whole childhood)*
Locked in my: _____ *(organ/ or whole being)*
Replace with opposite positive feelings of: _____

Part C: *I do a written forgiveness of the person who hurt me. (I surrender to God any need to punish).*
I now forgive _____ for causing me to suffer, and I ask him/ her to forgive me if I caused any pain. I forgive myself for holding these negative feelings.

Part D: *Sign and burn the document*

Read the document out-loud. <u>Sign and burn</u> it to facilitate releasing and removing retained negative feelings from your mind and body.

* * *

Example of a Written Release

Part A: *I write about my pain with a failed business.*

Part B: *I now release...*

Issue: *overwhelmed, ruined, destitute*
Due to: *my financial ruin*
Age: *from the last 5 years*
Locked: *in my whole being (and overloading into my mental body)*

Replace: *100% accepting what happened as I completely recover and start over again; 100% regaining my mental balance and positive thinking, and health.*

Part C / D:
Do the forgiveness/ Sign and burn the document.

In Part A you write about the issue you went through, and how you unconsciously reacted to this pain (write as many pages as it takes).

In Part B insert the feelings you probably went through (have an intelligent guess; the reprogramming will still happen).

In Part C write the appropriate forgiveness of whoever is involved in the issue.

In Part D sign and burn the document to release the programming.

* * *

Notes and Questions

(A muscle test is helpful if you know that tool. Otherwise, use your intuition and best educated guess.)

1. Ask: Do I have any intense feelings locked in my whole being that may be overloading into my mental body causing negative thinking?

Probable feelings -

_____

_____

_____

_____

_____

After identifying your negative feelings, apply them to the written release.

* * *

2. *Do I have Emotion-Organ balance?*

Do I have any emotions locked in discrete organs of my body interfering with my healing? If so, they also need releasing for greater healing. (See my prior books or Booklet #2.)

What emotions am I holding: fear, anger, sadness, humiliation, embarrassment, shame, guilt, heartbreak, despair, rejection, self-anger, self-pity, etc.?

_____

_____

_____

_____

* * *

3. *Other thoughts around this issue*

_____

_____

_____

* * *

Step 4 — Action Board

This method helps you organize and manage life stresses and worries.

* * *

David Viscott, M.D., used the phrase *Action Board* in a book on managing stress. He was a Pulitzer Prize winning psychiatrist and I highly recommend all of his books. He theorized that daily charting of major stresses on a black or white board or large cardboard prevents stress from overloading into organs causing health problems. I find this tool to be a powerful aid in stress management for neutralizing negative thoughts. You take some written action everyday, even if that action is to write that nothing can be done.

How to Proceed

1. Give each stress a name and place it on the chart for each day of the coming week(s):

By using such a chart, you challenge your mind to think more clearly than it ordinarily would. You are also organizing it and your intuition to find needed answers. An example:

Stress	*Monday*	*Tuesday*	*Wed...*

Money

- *budgeting*
- *creating*
- *other*

Relationships

- *love*
- *friend*
- *work*
- *other*

Work Stress

- *boss*
- *new job?*
- *my attitude?*

Other Stress

- *more education*
- *other*

2. Each day think of something you can do about the stress, and write it on the chart. For example, the phone number of someone you can call to seek help with that stress. Nothing may come to you, which happens, but do the discipline of reading and writing something on the chart everyday to reflect your decision: *not today, next week, not yet, later, etc.* (Do not write negative statements like: "It will never happen" or "My life is over" or "I'm a failure," etc.).

If you say negative phrases, or write them, you set yourself up to prolong that condition in your life.

* * *

3. Tomorrow think about it again. Rack your brain for some action you can take. Look at *each* stress item, think about it, and everyday write something on the chart: people, phone numbers, etc.

Sooner or later you will get a new idea. Ask a friend to help you with any new ideas. There is always something to do, so start mastering your worries. This definitely helps your mental balance and healing.

* * *

Notes and **Questions**

(A muscle test is helpful if you know that tool. Otherwise, use your intuition and best educated guess.)

* * *

1. Ask: Do I need an Action Board to organize my major worries and intense thinking?

If you are reading this booklet, you probably do need an Action Board, so write down your worries and start creating it.

My major worries:

_____

_____

_____

_____

_____

_____

* * *

2. Other thoughts around this issue

_____

_____

_____

▶ *Keeping stress information in your head does not resolve mental stress; in fact, it magnifies the stress and prevents healing. Writing about your mental stresses in a notebook is of little help. You must get your worries out of your head into plain view. Keep an Action Board on the wall, and write on it everyday.*

* * *

Step 5 — Behavioral Changes

You may need behavioral changes to lessen your mental stress and to enhance your healing.

* * *

This section deals with lessening the impact of mental stress on your mind and body. For example, it is your choice where you work and for whom you work. It may seem that you are stuck in a particular workplace with an unappreciative boss, but you owe it to yourself to do better and to find a more fulfilling work; likewise, for other choices you make like staying in a destructive relationship, or not educating yourself, etc.

If you need help in giving yourself permission to change or to remove yourself from a negative situation and to re-establish your mental balance, then the following three steps are useful:

A. Do Affirmations
B. Release Intense Negative Emotions
C. Appeal to God

A. Do Affirmations

* * *

For behavioral changes around mental balance revisit Step 2 and design an affirmation for your situation (said twenty-one times, twice daily, for two weeks):

Example: A Bad Work Situation

"I continue to give 100% effort as I explore all opportunities to find a fulfilling job and to stay in mental balance"

Example: A Bad Relationship

"I find the inner strength to leave this destructive relationship, to find refuge with family or friends and to stay in mental balance."

Or:

"I remain polite with my (mother, father, sibling, etc.) as I become non-reactive to their negativity and I stay in mental balance."

* * *

B. *Release Intense Negative Emotions*

* * *

For behavioral changes around mental balance, you need to release any *intense* negative emotions locked in your *whole being.* If stuck somewhere in your life, a toxic relationship, job, etc., search for and release the emotions you are feeling. Such feelings overload into your mental body causing negative thinking and ill-health.

Examples for a Written Release:

- *Fear, dread, or terror* (that I am stuck in this relationship; good things will never happen for me; I'm unqualified, useless, etc.)

- *Anger, rage, fury* (that…as above)

- *Unreal expectations* (that…as above)

- *Low self-esteem, worth, image, pride, etc.* (that…as above)

In the above examples, replace:

- *Fear, dread, or terror* with fearlessness, bravery, courage in believing there is a job for me, etc., and with mental balance

- *Anger, rage, and fury* with calm, peace, and tranquility as I take action, become more non-reactive to any negative situation, and with mental balance

- *Unreal expectations* with taking action, staying in reality, being happy living in the moment, and with mental balance

- *Low self-esteem, worth, image, pride, etc.,* with high self-esteem, etc., no matter what stress I have, and with mental balance

Examples for Releasing Intense Feelings:

Review the list on page 16, for your probable intense emotions, release them from your whole being, and replace them with the opposite positive feeling. (See the following example.)

_____

_____

Example of
Releasing Intense Emotions

Part A: *I write about my pain around not having a fulfilling job.*

Part B: *I now release …*
Issue: *fear, dread, and terror I will never find fulfilling work*
Due to: *my job ending*
Age: *from the last two years*
Locked: *in my whole being*
Replace: *100% accepting the situation; 100% fearlessness and bravery as this situation works out, and believing there is a better job for me, as I stay in mental balance.*

Part C/D:

    Do the forgiveness/Sign and burn the document.

C. *Appeal to God*

* * *

For behavioral changes around mental balance, an appeal to God may be appropriate. Affirm out-loud (twenty-one times, twice daily, for two weeks) something like:

"I co-create with God my highest opportunity for advancement and to finding fulfilling work as I stay in mental balance."

Or:

"I call upon God to help me maintain 100% mental balance and positive thinking in my relationship as it works out" *(or with my boss, or in another area of life).*

Or:

Apply these three steps to any other stress you have in your life.

* * *

Notes and Questions

(A muscle test is helpful if you know that tool. Otherwise, use your intuition and best educated guess.)

* * *

1. Ask: Do I need to change my behavior to regain mental balance and positive thinking?

If yes, then look closely at your life, ask your loved ones about it, and take some action.

My possible negative behaviors:

_____

_____

* * *

2. Ask: Do I need to change my job, employment, career, etc., to lessen my mental stress? If so, how should I proceed?

_____

_____

* * *

3. Ask: Do I need to confront a personal issue with someone, a parent, sibling, friend, etc., to lessen my mental stress?

_____

_____

* * *

4. Other thoughts around this issue:

_____

_____

* * *

Step 6 — Adrenal Hypoglycemia Recovery

Adrenal hypoglycemia (low blood sugar) must be resolved since it causes more mental stress.

* * *

Low blood sugar is a complex subject discussed in the earlier books; *adrenal hypoglycemia* is one important cause of negative thinking.

The adrenal glands, situated on the kidneys, make over one hundred hormones, adrenal under-activity producing a common low blood sugar condition that is often due to the wide-spread abuse and reaction to white sugar products (sodas, cakes, cookies, ice cream, etc.). Those of you having a severe form of hypoglycemia also become sensitive to fruits and carbohydrates. Genetically weak adrenal glands aggravate this condition and anyone with severe mental stress is likely to have this problem.

Stress, exhaustion, nutritional deficiencies, and chemical, metal, or free radical toxicity in the body are factors commonly found in adrenal problems.

Common symptoms of adrenal hypoglycemia:

- Fatigue
- Fainting
- Headaches
- Dilated pupils
- Visual problems
- Cold intolerance
- Menses problems
- Failure, self-failure
- Loss of motivation
- Poor healing ability
- Sex organ problems
- Low blood pressure
- Self: anger, rage, fury
- Knee pain or weakness
- Mood swings or depression
- Neck, mid- and low back pain
- Mental stress and negative thinking
- Bone, joint, teeth, gums, skin, and connective tissue problems

▶ *There are two-sides to adrenal hypoglycemia: one that it causes mental stress and negative thinking; the other, that mental stress causes adrenal hypoglycemia!*

* * *

Adrenal Gland Treatment

1. Nutrition

Be sure to follow the food advice in *Step 1* regarding the nurturing of the nerves responsible for your thinking. Keep taking them until your adrenal gland symptoms are resolved. Also take the following products, two capsules, twice daily with food, for one month, then once daily for another month:

Adrenal Extract or Concentrate; or
Saw Palmetto Herb (if vegetarian)

*** *

2. Negative Emotion Release

Use the written release (page 18) and write about any memories involving the following emotions:

- Failure
- Self-failure
- Self: anger, rage, and fury

Replace these negatives with:
- Success and self-success
- Self: calm, peace, tranquility

Most people go through such feelings in childhood, often from feeling anger or failure (around a parent, teacher, or a situation), the feelings then *automatically turn against ourselves.* We are then prone to feeling anger, failure, etc., *without* any external stimulation. We apply the emotion and behavior to ourselves! This situation usually happens from *not* feeling loved enough in childhood. Did you receive such positive reinforcement from parents?

* * *

Example: Releasing the Adrenal Cause of Mental Stress

Part A: *I write about the lack of accomplishment in my life.*

Part B: *I now release …*

Issue: *failure (and self-failure)*
Due to: *my business (or relationship) failure*
Age: *from the last seven years*
Locked: *in my adrenal glands*

Replace: *100% accepting what happened, as I recover and never give up; 100% knowing I am successful (and self-successful) in God's eyes and that is what is important; 100% mental balance, positive thinking, and adrenal balance.*

Part C / D: *Do the forgiveness/Sign and burn the document.*

---

* * *

Notes and Questions

(A muscle test is helpful if you know that tool. Otherwise, use your intuition and best educated guess.)

* * *

1. Ask: Do I have any of the previously mentioned symptoms?

You may only have a few of those symptoms, but still be suffering with this condition, so do the recommended treatment.

* * *

2. Ask: Do I have any other cause of low blood sugar?

You could also have dysfunction of the liver, pituitary, or pancreas, any of which cause hypoglycemia and complicate your ability to master mental stress. (If so, read about such issues in my prior books, work through them and resolve these conditions.)

Dr. Lloyd Stenbeck

My possible causes of low blood sugar:

_____

_____

_____

* * *

3. Other thoughts around this issue:

_____

_____

_____

* * *

Step 7 — DNA or a Spiritual Cause of Mental Stress

You may have a DNA or life lesson factor causing mental stress and interfering with your healing.

***

1. The DNA Factor

A DNA factor may affect your mental balance and cause negative thinking. Some of you have a genetic inheritance situation coming from a parent. You may have inherited from their DNA a predisposition to mental stress (or to being neurotic or having some other condition). This is relatively common so look carefully at the behaviors of your family members. Their DNA is also in you, to some degree. If your brain and nervous system has this inclination then after accomplishing the prior *Steps* you are ready to address the DNA factor.

The need for re-programming of damaged DNA comes from recent research in cell biology, and this exciting new science may lead to new directions in the medical treatment of cancer and other diseases. Holistic suggestions given here help with this re-programming.

Important Research in Cell Biology

Research published in the esteemed science journal *Nature* shows that although the gene pool is mostly stable and unchanging throughout life, about 1.5% of our DNA is fluid, dynamic, and changeable. This genetic aspect, called the *epigenome*, means "in addition to genetics"; it functions to turn genes on or off, for better or worse, for healing or not, contributing to your mental disturbances, whether slight or gross.

▶ *This research showed that severe stress, fatty diets, and toxin exposure (smoking, etc.), cause the epigenome to work against our health.*

The stability of your healthy gene expression is due to a metabolic process known as *"DNA methylation."* Many substances, known to alter this process, have a positive or negative effect on your healthy gene expression.

Positive Factors Influencing the Epigenome — by Kanherkar and others

A few extracts follow on this subject from, *Frontiers in Cell and Developmental Biology*.

They point out how negative substances affect the epigenome, like: alcohol, smoking, heavy metals, pharmaceuticals, and recreational drugs, which then may initiate toxic disease processes like cancer, arthritis, cardiovascular disease, etc.

Scientific research has demonstrated that alternative medicine (Ayurveda, naturopathy, massage, etc.), has a positive affect on the epigenome and healthy DNA methylation.

Kanherkar states:

Some of the beneficial influences listed are exercise, microbiome (beneficial intestinal bacteria), and alternative medicine whereas harmful influences include exposure to toxic chemicals and drugs of abuse…with the help of extensive research in the field, we might be able to steer these influences in a positive way.

And on maintaining healthy DNA methylation:

Dietary folate (folic acid) present in a variety of green vegetables including broccoli, zucchini, Brussels sprouts, green beans and spinach participates in maintaining a healthy DNA methylation profile and even *reverses* accrued damage.

It has also been reported that ginger, curcumin (from turmeric) and anthocyanins (phytochemicals and pigmented plants) fight free radicals thereby enhancing DNA methylation and healing.

The research in this area is extensive, very technical, with many scientists being excited about this field of study. The first medication to help the epigenome maintain DNA methylation is now available.

▶ *In this booklet, the question is how to manipulate this DNA factor in your favor. Holistic healers utilize your healing consciousness, the inherent power of the mind to help reprogram the epigenome for your healing.*

I have seen little research to support the holistic discussion in this Step, other than vague references to the positive influences of psychology and alternative medicine in maintaining DNA methylation. The holistic approach to preventing and healing DNA damage, preventing disease, and enhancing healing is evolving, and hopefully the method presented here will contribute to your healing.

Scientific validation of the power your *conscious mind* has over enhancing positive epigenome activity may, or may not, be in our future, but holistic doctors have been exploring this aspect of re-programming for years.

* * *

Re-programming Damaged DNA

If you may have a family DNA factor affecting your mental balance then the nutrition in *Step 1* is very important. Take the nutrition for a longer period of time: for *two* months and then once daily for another month. Then take them three times weekly for maintenance.

▶ *Note that this booklet only discusses Mental issues, but the DNA reprogramming may be applied to any healing problem.*

It is advantageous to do this re-programming even if you don't particularly relate to it.

A. Spoken DNA Re-programming
and
B. Written DNA Re-programming

* * *

A. <u>Spoken</u> (DNA Re-programming)

Choose one of these affirmations and say it out-loud, twenty-one times, *once* daily, for <u>four</u> weeks:

"I <u>consciously command</u> that my damaged DNA be returned to its original perfect condition, as I return to 100% mental balance."

Or:

"I <u>consciously command</u> that my damaged DNA be returned to its original perfect condition, and any predisposition I have to being mentally stressed (or to any other mental disturbance) is now cancelled."

Or:

*"I <u>consciously command</u>, **in God's name** that my damaged DNA be returned to its original perfect condition, etc.*

* * *

An example follows of the type of written release needed to reprogram your damaged DNA.

B. _Written_ (DNA Re-programming)

Part A: *I write about my mental stress symptoms and how they affect me.*

Part B: *I now reprogram…*

Issue: *My _damaged DNA_ that causes _my vulnerability to mental stress_ (or to other mental conditions)*

Due to: *my genetics, bad diet, stress, etc.*
Age: *my whole life from conception*
Locked: *in my _whole being_*

Replace: *I _consciously command_ that my _DNA be returned to its original perfect condition;_ and 100% _mental balance and positive thinking_.*

Part C / D:
Do the forgiveness/ Sign and burn the document.

The holistic DNA re-programming represents an act of your conscious mind. Some people are born with a very strong mental body and are more able to naturally command and accomplish such re-programming and healing. The rest of us have to work harder. This Step seeks to help you with that goal.

Notes and Questions

(A muscle test is helpful if you know that tool. Otherwise, use your intuition and best educated guess.)

* * *

1. Ask: Do I have a damaged DNA factor predisposing me to being mentally stressed (or to having some other mental problem)?

This is relatively common so look carefully at the behaviors of your family members (parent, sibling, relative, etc.). Does someone show evidence of mental stress or instability? If so, some of this damaged DNA is present in you.

My family DNA problems (re-mental balance):

_____

_____

* * *

2. Other thoughts around this issue

_____

* * *

2. *The Life Lesson Factor*

Skip this section if you are not spiritual or do not believe in life lessons, soul projects, or in your spiritual evolution. You need to believe in a creator or a higher power to relate to this material. [See Booklet #3 for more information on Spiritual Balance and the integrity of your God relationship, and for the factors that interfere with it.]

* * *

A soul project, in the context of this booklet, is a life lesson, usually a negative situation, something that as a soul you chose to go through for evolutionary purposes. If you have this aspect, then after accomplishing the prior Steps you are now ready to identify the life lesson. In this booklet, you are particularly looking for the lesson that applies to your mental stress vulnerability or to a more complex mental disorder.

Any of the following projects may impact on your mental balance and positive thinking. If you don't relate to any of them think about some other personal life lesson that fits your life experiences. If you identify with an issue, then do the following re-programming through spoken and written releases.

Examples of Soul Projects or Life Lessons

Your individuality ensures that there are an infinite number of life lesson possibilities, common examples being:

- Feeling separated from God
- Not accepting that God controls my life
- Not having close loving communion with family, friends, others
- Having antisocial or sociopathic habits (sexual, stealing, lying…)
- Not being a devoted, loving, honest, trustworthy partner or spouse
- Needing to try and accomplish something important for the evolution of mankind
- Not being accepting of my life, because my talents are unrecognized
- Not accepting that even with my meager accomplishments, I am a beloved of God
- Not accepting my financial status, right now, as being exactly what it is supposed to be for my evolution
- Having a "runaway mind" or negative thinking, or unable to be positive
- Your choices

Re-programming a Life Lesson

Identify a life lesson and then do:

A. *Spoken* Life Lesson Reprogramming
and
B. *Written* Life Lesson Reprogramming

* * *

A. *Spoken* Life Lesson Reprogramming

Affirm this affirmation out-loud, twenty-one times, once daily, for four weeks:

"I command that my Life Lesson of.......
...

now be released from every cell of my being, and replaced with the opposite positive programming of
...

and with 100% mental balance, positive thinking, and accomplishing my life lesson."

* * *

B. <u>Written</u> Life Lesson Re-programming

<u>**Part A:**</u> *I write about my life lessons of...*

<u>**Part B:**</u> *I now release...*

Issue: *My life lesson of* _____
Due to: *the unhappiness of my life*
Age: *my whole life from conception*
Locked: *in my <u>whole being</u>*

Replace: *100% <u>commanding</u> that my life lesson of* _____ *be completed and replaced with* _____; *and with 100% <u>mental balance</u> and <u>positive thinking</u>.*

<u>**Part C / D:**</u>
Do the forgiveness/Sign and burn the document.

* * *

Notes and Questions

(A muscle test is helpful if you know that tool. Otherwise, use your intuition and best educated guess.)

* * *

1. Ask: What are my probable soul projects or life lessons?

_____

_____

_____

Do the appropriate reprogramming.

* * *

2. Other thoughts around this issue

_____

_____

_____

* * *

Summary

The simple Steps presented here help you become more positive in your thinking than you have ever been. For most people, doing these Steps will automatically make you a more positive and healthier person. Check my webpage for more holistic self-healing information:

DrStenbeck.net

You can always email me, from the website, if you require more help with your healing.

I hope you have found this Booklet useful for your healing. If you have, be sure to follow up with Booklet #2 on clearing negative emotions from your mind and body, replacing them with their opposite positive feelings and behaviors, and with becoming healthier:

"Mastering Positive Feelings for Health"

Appendix

Further Reading

Alexander F: _Psychosomatic Medicine_, Norton, NY, 1965. Fine introduction to the psychological aspects of disease.

Antonovsky A: _Health, Stress and Coping_, Jansey Bass, 1979. A good account of stress and disease.

Cheraskin E, Ringsdorf WM: _Psycho-Dietetics_, Stein and Day Publishing Company, NY, 1975. Nicely describes the place of nutrients in treating psychological disorders.

Dorian B: Abberations in Lymphatic Sub-Populations and Functions During Psychological Stress, _Clin Exper Immuno_ 50:132-138, 1982. Documents the stress, neural and hormonal aspects of immune suppression, and disease.

Fredericks C: Psychonutrition, Grosset and Dunlap, 1955. Discusses the natural treatment of mental disorders.

Goldman D, Gurin J (Ed's): *Higher Self-Body Medicine*, Consumer Reports Books, NY, 1993. Excellent review of the field, with references.

Graham, DT, Stevenson I: *Physiological Basis of Medical Practice*: Disease as a response to life stress, Harper and Row, NY, 1963. Good discussion of stress and disease.

Hawkins D, Pauling L: *Orthomolecular Psychiatry*, Reading, San Francisco, 1973. Classic book on the nutritional treatment of psychiatric problems.

Hay L: *Heal Your Life*, Hay House, Carlsbad, CA 1986. An essential aid to forgiveness and self-forgiveness; organ and emotion issues and remedial affirmations.

Holmes TH, Rahe RH: The Social Readjustment Rating Scale, *J Psychosom Res* 11:213-218, 1967. Research on the significant impact of stress on health.

Holmes TH, Rahe R, and others: *The Nose.* An Experimental Study of Reactions within the Nose in Human Subjects during varying Life Experiences, Thomas, Springfield. Shows how thinking of stressful events causes tissue damage.

Kanherkar, Bhatia, Csoka: Epigenetics Across the Human Lifespan, *Frontiers in Cell and Developmental Biology,* September 2014. Presents a comprehensive review of the subject with many references.

Lewis C, and others: *The Psychoimmunology of Cancer,* Oxford University Press, NY, 1994. Hundreds of references on the psychological relationships to disease.

Masek K, and others: Past, Present and Future of Psycho-neuroimmunology, *Toxicology* 142, 179-188, 2000. The influence of the mind on disease.

Maxwell J: *The Eye/Body Connection,* Warne Books, 1979. Comprehensive account of iris analysis in healing, and stress management (based on interviews with Dr. Stenbeck and others).

Metal'nikov S: Role Des Reflexes Conditionnels Dans l'immuite, *Ann Inst Pasteur,* 1926. Earliest study demonstrating effects of psychology on the immune response.

Newbold H: *Meganutrients for Your Nerves,* Peter H. Wyden, NY, 1975. The orthomolecular nutritional approach to healing.

Oyle I: *The Healing Mind*, Pocket Books, NY, 1976. Classic book on mental healing.

Pauling L: Orthomolecular Psychiatry, *Sci* 160:265-271, 1968. The Nobel prize winner's work on using nutrition for healing the mind.

Ponder K: *The Healing Secret of The Ages*, DeVorss and Company, CA, 1966. One of Ponder's many excellent books on mental affirmations in healing.

Selye H: The Story of the Adaptation Syndrome, Montreal: *Acta Inc Med Publ*, 1952. Discusses organ reactions to stress. Selye wrote many excellent books and scientific articles on stress.

Selye H: *The Stress of Life*, McGraw Hill, NY, 1978. Essential reading on understanding how the physiology of stress damages the body.

Siegel B: Love, *Medicine and Miracles*, Harper and Row, NY, 1986. Popular book on integrating the mind and healing.

Simeons A: *Man's Presumptuous Brain*, EP Dutton and Co., Inc., USA, 1960. A brilliant, ground-breaking book on psychosomatic medicine.

Simonton O: *Getting Well Again*, JP Tarcher, Inc., 1978. A classic new age healing work on mind/body integration.

Tache J, and others: *Cancer, Stress and Death*, Plenum Press, NY, 1979. Correlation of stress events with disease.

Viscott D: *The Viscott Method*, Houghton Mifflin Company, Boston, 1984. Manual for mastering the stress of life. One of his many useful books.

Watson G: *Nutrition and Your Higher Self*, Bantam, 1971. Fascinating account of nutrition and brain function.

Yogananda P: *Where There is Light*, Self-Realization Fellowship Press, Los Angeles, 1988. Inspirational Indian saint's work on mastering the stress of life.

* * *

Finding Holistic Doctors

To contact a holistic doctor who does muscle testing try:

> *www.appliedkinesiology.org*
> Or: *www.touchforhealth.us*
> Or: *www.icakusa.com*
> Or: Contact your local chiropractic association and ask for referrals to doctors doing applied kinesiology or muscle testing.

* * *

Contacting Dr. Stenbeck

For further information, or to comment on this book, or to receive some free advice on any *one* health issue from a holistic viewpoint, see his web site: *DrStenbeck.net*

* * *

Notes